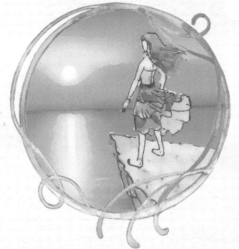

The Beginners' 10 Step Guide to the Sexual Universe

This book is not intended as medical advice. Its intent is educational. Please consult a health professional should
the need for one be indicated.

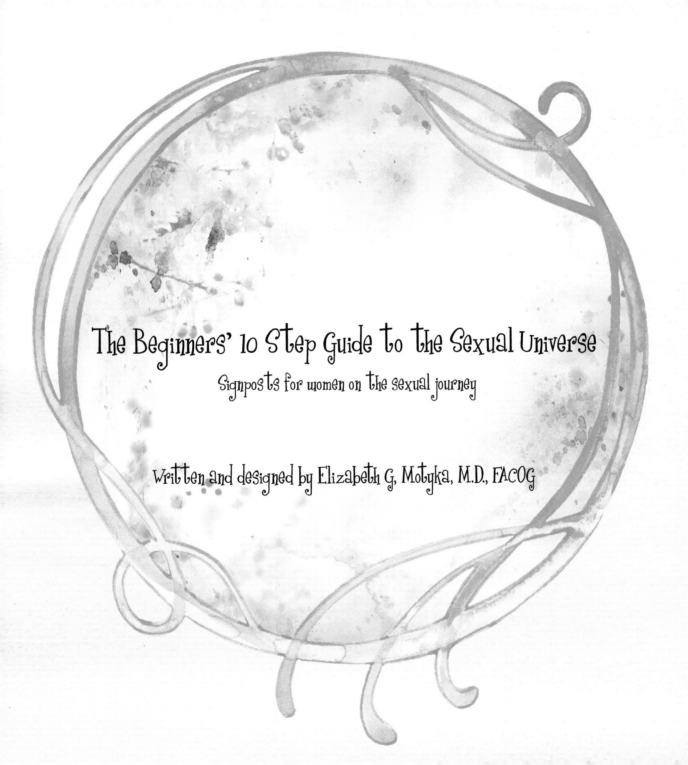

The Beginners' 10 Step Guide to the Sexual Universe

Signposts for women on the sexual journey

Written and designed by Elizabeth G. Motyka, M.D., FACOG

Set your life on fire, Seek those who fan the flames

-Rumi

For our daughters

Becoming a Sexual Being

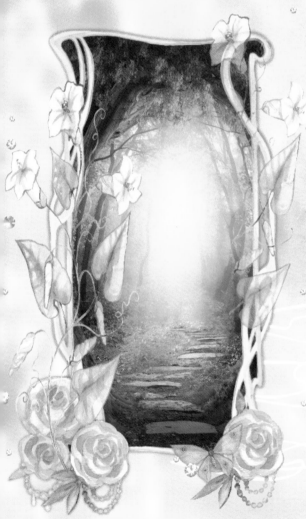

Deciding to have sex is an important decision. Becoming a sexual being is a process that evolves over a lifetime. This process starts with your first feeling of attraction, and from there, as you learn to give and receive pleasure, you grow with each new experience. Kissing, touching, desire, oral sex, orgasm, vaginal intercourse, intimacy, and ecstasy are all pleasures that are part of becoming a sexual being. Really all the parts of the human experience that have to do with desire for sexual exploration and gratification, acceptance by others, self-acceptance, and relationship development are part of becoming a sexual being.

When you have sex for the first time, you cross a threshold from not knowing to knowing. The concept of losing your virginity is outdated and harmful: there is no "thing" that can be lost, given, or taken, there is only knowledge to be gained. There is no medical condition that correlates with virginity and there is no capacity to become impure. Rather, as you grow with each encounter you mature and expand your abilities.

First sexual experiences can color a person's feelings about sex for years to come. The right information can prevent confusion and pain. Planning can foster enjoyment and pleasure. If you are new to sexual experiences, then the following ideas can help you decide if the time is right for you. If you are ready to start this journey, this book can help you have safe and enjoyable sex from the beginning. If you have been abstinent for some time, it can help you begin again. These ten steps can help anyone become a more conscious and confident sexual being, and in time blossom into their full sexual potential.

Broadly speaking, any activity, where a person gives or takes sexual gratification, is sexual activity.

1

1. Discover when you are ready

All sexual play needs to be consensual. You need to decide for yourself what is okay for you. It is important not to feel pressured by your peers or your partner, but wait until the time feels right whether that be after a few dates, several months, or on your honeymoon. **Your partner should never make you feel like it is now or never.** Instead, be clear about why you want to have sex with another person and weigh the pros and cons carefully for yourself. Ideally, you should have a partner with similar goals for the experience. People's goals for sex are often very different. For example, some people are motivated because they are looking to experience increased intimacy or closeness with a partner. Other motivations for sex might be to experience pleasure, creativity, control, relief from stress, or conquest (the winning of sexual favors from multiple partners.) So, discover what is motivating your partner and see how it fits with your own wishes and needs. **Despite what media commonly suggests, a woman does not need to have sex to fulfil her partner's needs, but can wait until she is ready to have a shared pleasurable experience.**

Physical attraction is a powerful sexual motivator, but not usually enough for a really good sexual experience. Early on in relationships, attraction is a strong physical sexual turn-on, especially when you are young and your hormones are actively driving sexual desire. Whether you act on physical attraction or not is a conscious choice you make. Having someone "like you" in itself is not a foundation for a good sexual relationship. **For sex to be meaningful it can't just be a receptive act, but rather you both need to actively decide if you know, like, and respect each other well enough to connect in a deep way.**

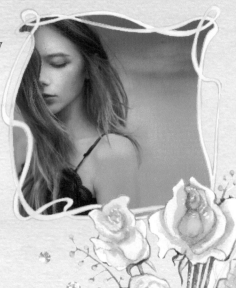

Sexual intimacy with another person involves opening yourself up to a person with your body, mind, heart, and spirit. Taking this risk has potentially positive or negative outcomes. Physically, your partner may touch you intimately or see you naked and vulnerable. You may be risking parenthood with that person. Mentally, you share your intimate thoughts, beliefs, and ideas. You risk your reputation. Emotionally, sex increases your vulnerability. It is natural to open our hearts to our sexual partners and each time you reveal your feelings, you risk a little more. Spiritually, you have the opportunity to connect with each other on a deeper and more profound level. This connection can uplift you or bring you down. Jeering or insulting comments from a former lover do not just cause heartbreak; they make you feel as if you have been put down or "slimed." A true spiritual connection, however can lead to love, joy, and ecstasy.

The key to discovering when you are ready is getting to know your partner well enough to feel attracted to their character as well as their face and body. Are they trustworthy, do they have integrity, and do they care about your well being? When you share your thoughts and feelings do they listen and appreciate without judging? Do they risk revealing themselves to you? Trust your intuition; you will know if the chemistry and timing are right. You are considering letting another person enter your physical, intellectual, emotional, and spiritual life and that act should be done with care.

Journaling prompts
The sexual journey is one of self discovery. Writing in a journal is one way to help you discover your thoughts and feelings. Throughout this book you will find questions that prompt you to journal.

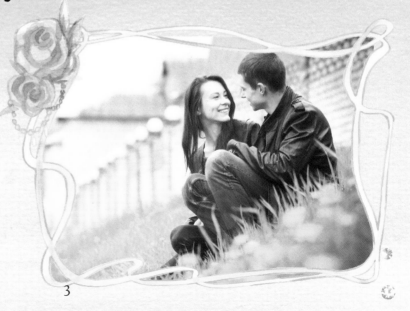

What are your thoughts and feelings about starting the sexual journey?

What are your motivations and those of your partner ?

Do you feel ready to make an independent, conscious, decision (give consent)?

3

2. Follow your own path

Society, culture, and religious groups seek to define sexuality, often with negative and confusing judgments and messages. Whether their prohibitions stem from a fear of pleasure or a need to control sexuality, deciding what you think about these messages can be complicated. From a scientific standpoint, when experienced safely and in moderation, physical pleasure, emotional joy, and spiritual connection do not cause harm.

It is natural for couples who are attracted to each other to want to try different sexual activities. Included in this is the freedom to decide which gender(s) you identify with and which gender(s) you are attracted to. As you first become sexually aware, you may notice your feelings about attraction vary based on experiences and depending on the individual partner you are with. You may find yourself attracted to members of the same or the opposite sex. This is normal. The steps in this book work for straight, lesbian or bisexual couples.

Learning what feels good to you and your partner and giving and receiving pleasure in a safe space are natural, human, and life affirming activities. They are not something you should ever feel ashamed of. I have found in my medical practice that societal and religious definitions of how sex "should be" and what is considered wrong, immoral or impure, can cause emotional and sexual problems. Shaming the physical can lead to repressed emotions, numbness, sexual impotence, anger and sexual violence. Ultimately, it is your body, your decision, and your journey of sexual expression.

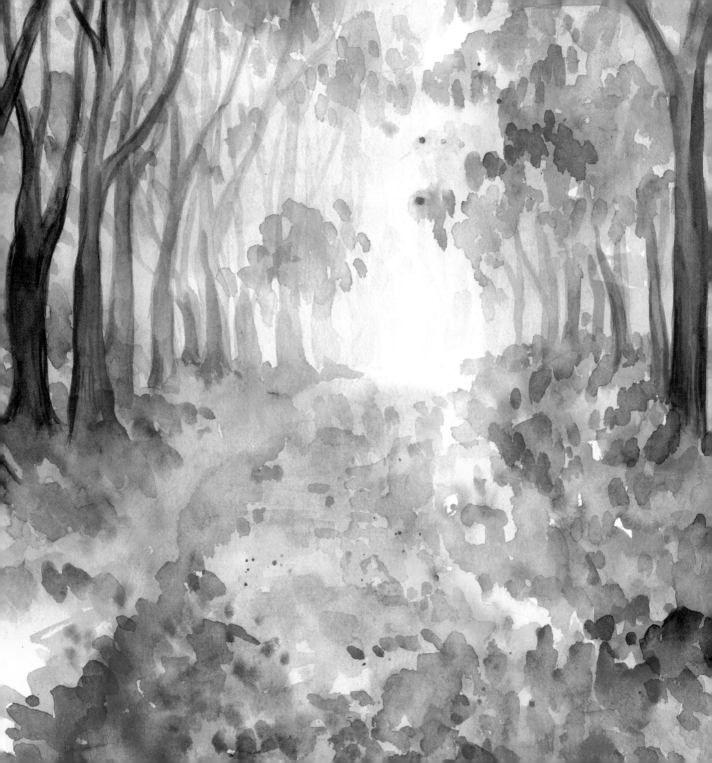

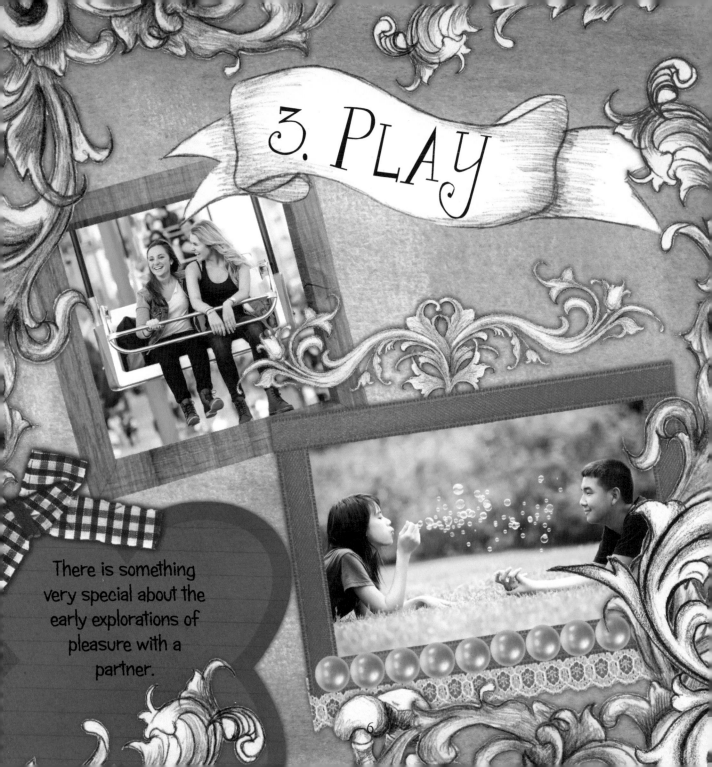

3. PLAY

There is something very special about the early explorations of pleasure with a partner.

Take lots of time to get to know each other physically and emotionally. Ideally as your relationship grows, each person learns what feels good to the other. Before having vaginal intercourse, get to know each other's body and responses.

You can begin to get to know a partner while others are present or close by. Dates with other friends or on your own at an ice rink, restaurant, or movie theater provide an opportunity to check out what you have in common. Even if you know your partner very well, it is still fun to start slow by learning what feels good to each other. Lots of couples learn by "making out ." Kissing. french kissing (tongue touching while kissing) massaging or fondling each other while fully dressed will reveal if there is chemistry and trust between you. The lips, neck, ears, eyelids, hair, hands, shoulders, breasts, back, thighs, and feet are full of pleasure receptors ready for you both to explore. These areas, which are also known as erogenous zones, are parts of the body that when stroked or kissed can result in arousal (being turned on) and sensations of delight. Time spent kissing, touching, licking, tapping, sucking, nibbling, stroking, looking deeply at, and massaging each other's nongenital erogenous zones is a fun and pleasurable part of sex. Sexual play that does not involve genital touch and vaginal penetration is sometimes known as "outercourse."

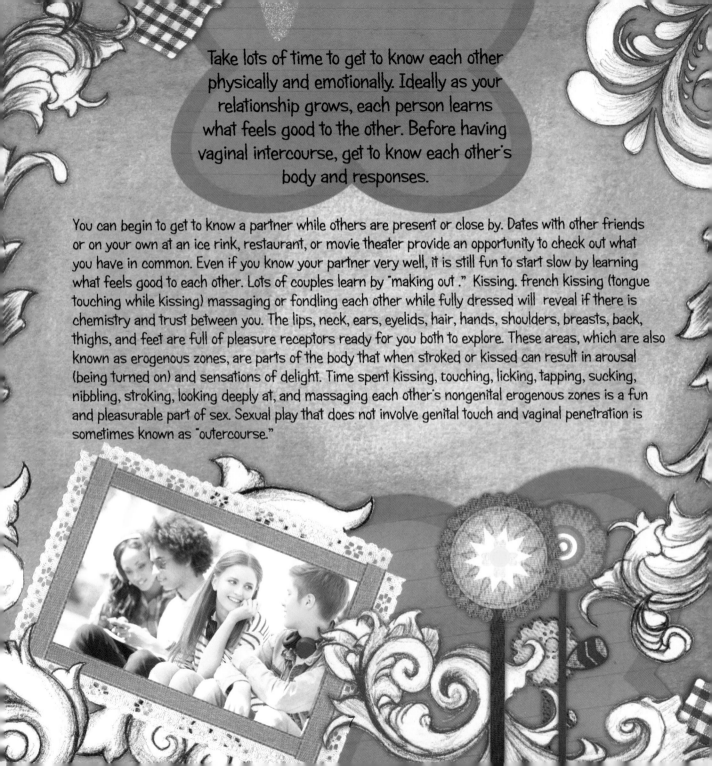

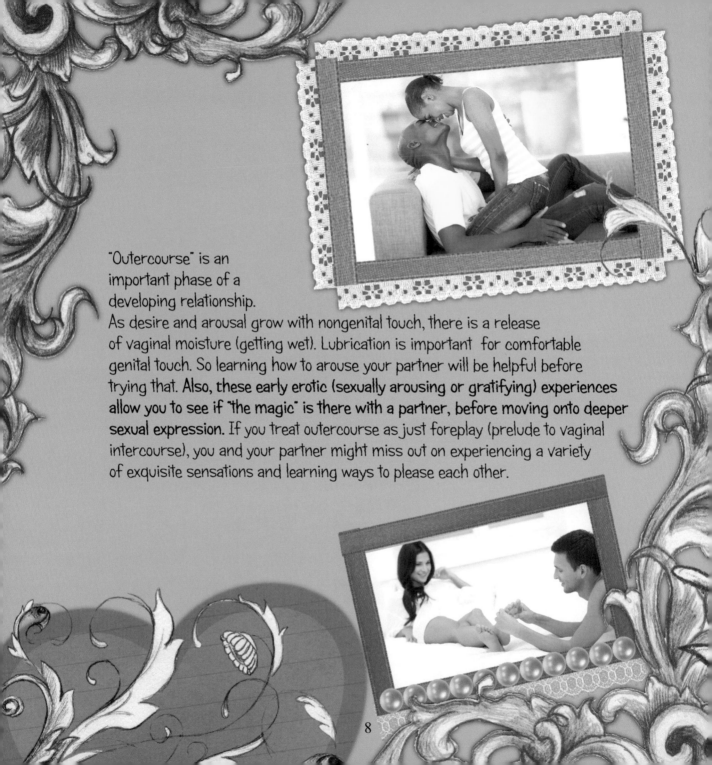

"Outercourse" is an important phase of a developing relationship. As desire and arousal grow with nongenital touch, there is a release of vaginal moisture (getting wet). Lubrication is important for comfortable genital touch. So learning how to arouse your partner will be helpful before trying that. Also, these early erotic (sexually arousing or gratifying) experiences allow you to see if "the magic" is there with a partner, before moving onto deeper sexual expression. If you treat outercourse as just foreplay (prelude to vaginal intercourse), you and your partner might miss out on experiencing a variety of exquisite sensations and learning ways to please each other.

Genital (sexual organ) contact and orgasm tend to involve more letting go of control and a deeper sharing of what turns you on. Nongenital touch will allow you to "feel the wanting" without risking so much. **Desire and longing are as much a part of the erotic experience as climax and resolution.** Spending time in play and exploration, will deepen your relationship and your desire for your partner. Once your relationship progresses past this stage and into deeper sexual intimacy, it is difficult to go back to more innocent play. So take your time and enjoy this phase. Instant gratification may seem appealing, but allowing the desire to build, be savored, and unfold more gradually can create a more erotic, satisfying, and powerful experience. In the early days of relationships, we often have fun by going on dates and discovering things we mutually share or enjoy. We are often most open to exploring and trying new things, so this is an ideal time to fully explore outercourse. **In these early days, we often present "our best self"** to our partner. Time spent playing together eventually allows you to express your "true self" to each other. Accepting who each other truly is and accepting your differences builds trust. Trust allows you to know when it is safe and time to continue on your sexual journey.

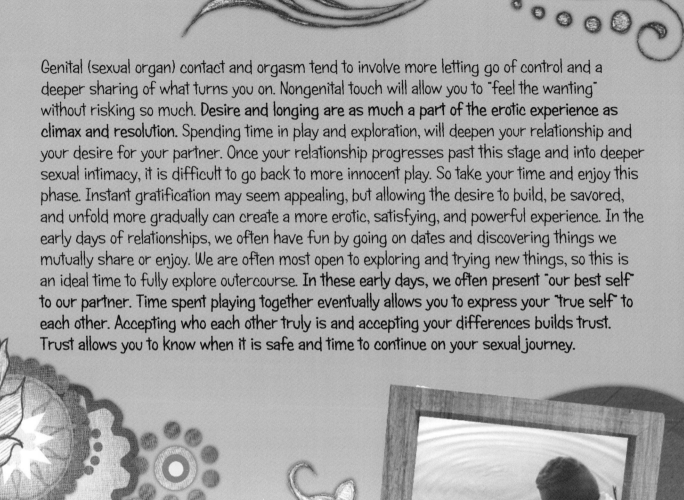

♀ 4. Get to know your inner "Venus"

After puberty, as your sex hormones increase, you start to become sexually aware and develop an individual sexual style. Your inner "Venus" (sexual self) is composed of what you find attractive, your way of attracting partners, how you find fulfillment on your journey, and what issues you might have or problems you might encounter. Sex is a multidimensional experience, involving the body, heart, mind, spirit. Your approach will combine these aspects in a unique way and will develop over time. Understanding one another's personal roads to fulfillment, inclusive of turn-ons and roadblocks, is good way to establish sexual intimacy.

Sexual styles vary from person to person. The body centered Venus may be very physical in his/her approach to sexuality; their focus is on the earthier or grounded experiences. Other more mind centered individuals love to connect through shared ideas. Opening the mind and imagination may make their desire hum. Sharing beauty and harmony may be the pathway that fulfills the romantic Venus. Passionate individuals may be turned on by more heart opening experiences. A person with this sexual mode may be hot, playful, or adventurous. Creative expression may be what brings them joy in bed. You may be, or you may meet partners where sexual satisfaction is triggered by playing with the balance of control and vulnerability. With this path, it is important to pay attention to the balance or imbalance of power in the relationship and make sure you are comfortable with the sharing of decision making. Mutual respect of boundaries and clear communication can facilitate safe connection. For others sexual bonding is about spiritual connection. Being able to feel linked to their partner intuitively by a look across a crowded room or gazing into their partner's eyes and breathing together are ways more mystical Venus can be expressed.

What do you know about what turns you on ? Check out the Venus Quiz on the next 3 pages to give you some ideas. Use the quiz as a way to get to know yourself. You can circle or make a list in your journal of the things that reflect you, that interest you, or that you see, or would like to see in a partner. Take a look at the road blocks that fall under your type(s). How can you avoid falling into those traps?

Your inner "Venus" Quiz

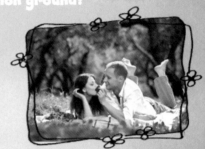

The body, emotion, mind and spirit centered types each have three inner Venus styles. Do you resonate with one or do you recognize yourself in a combination of these styles below? What about your partner? Where do you share common ground?

BODY CENTERED TYPE

- 1. Your road to fulfillment requires sensual pleasures, creature comforts, serenity, nature, and a slow pace.
- Your ideal date might include: backrubs, music, or a picnic in a garden or park.
- Your possible roadblocks to connection include: laziness, getting stuck in a rut, and practicing denial.

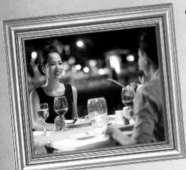

- 2. For you to find fulfillment you need a relationship that helps you be the best person you can be and one where you support your partner reach their highest potential. You like to be "working on" the relationship. Whether you like sophistication or simplicity, you will find pleasure in cultivating wholeness and perfection.
- Your ideal date might include: talking about your relationship at a restaurant with impeccable service, or learning to dance flawlessly together.
- Your possible roadblocks to connection include: perfectionism, nagging, being controlling, worrying, overworking, and insecurity.

- Your road to fulfillment depends upon commitment, loyalty, maturity, or working together on a mission.
- Your ideal date might be: going on an all day hike or climb, building a habitat for humanity house together, or eating in your favorite place once a week after a class you are taking together.
- Your possible roadblocks to connection include being: bossy, overly serious, stoic, or inflexible. You can suffer from a fear of trusting others.

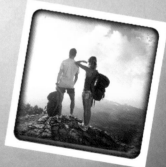

EMOTION CENTERED TYPE

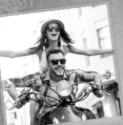

- 1. You can find your road to fulfillment by being direct, not playing games, feeling passion, and being able to speak your mind. You may enjoy a faster pace.
- Your ideal date likely involves taking a little risk... riding a rollercoaster at the fair, white water rafting, or going together to a protest march.
- Your possible roadblocks to connection include: being hot headed or fearful. These intense emotions can lead to bullying, impatience, exaggerating problems, or hardening your heart to your partner in an attempt to suppress your feelings.
    - 2. Your road to fulfillment requires being appreciated, being creative together, "falling in love," being treated like "a queen for a day," and being playful.
    - On your ideal date you are the center of your partner's attention. If you get dressed up, your partner notices and lets you know she/he likes it. You go out for dinner and all your jokes are laughed at and your conversation brings delight. You feel special.
    - Your possible roadblocks to connection include: insecurity, being self-centered, the tendency to try to overshadow others, and the compulsive need for approval.
- 3. For you to feel fulfilled you need meaningful adventures, giving and receiving big, noticeable gestures of affection or generosity. You like to feel that life is good.
- An ideal date might include going away for the weekend to visit a new place, treating your partner and a group of friends to front row seats at a concert.
- Your possible roadblocks to connection include: getting caught up in appearances or popularity, being self-righteous or opinionated, having poor boundaries. You suffer if you feel you are being starved for affection.

MIND CENTERED TYPE

- 1. For fulfillment you need to be heard, to be curious, to have novel experiences, to investigate things that are interesting.
- Your ideal date is to see a popular new show and then spend time after in clever, witty, flirty conversation about it. You may enjoy learning and doing new dance steps. Playing cards can be fun for you too.
- Your possible roadblocks to connection include: boredom, playing mind-games, defensiveness, restlessness, and nervousness.
- 2. For you to experience fulfillment you must have harmony, peace, and beauty. You need to be cherished.
- On an ideal date you like to be careful with your physical appearance. You might like to visit an art museum or a beautiful garden. You might like to take a romantic walk in the moonlight.
- Your possible roadblocks to connection include: being wishy-washy or co-dependent, and attempting to avoid conflict (to keep the peace).

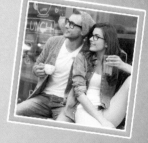

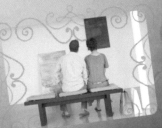

- 3. Your road to satisfaction or fulfillment takes innovation, freedom in relationship, and being unconventional.
- Your ideal date might include trying something out of the mainstream: anything from listening to alternative music, visiting an innovative exhibit at a museum, to a progressive political rally. You might like attending a reading, lecture, or performance if you get a chance to discuss your ideas or impressions with your partner.
- Your possible roadblocks to connection include being: distant, removed, or alienated. If you are forced to conform to cultural norms or feel you are being controlled, you will not be happy.

SPIRIT CENTERED TYPE

- 1. For fulfillment in relationships, you need someone to be sensitive to your feelings. You thrive on gentleness, giving and receiving nurturing, safety, nesting, loyalty and being openly cared for.
- Your ideal date might be a private dinner at home or maybe heading to a favorite bar where you are a regular. You might enjoy a day at the beach that includes lots of small touches and gestures of affection.
- Your possible roadblocks to connection include being: sulky, overly sensitive, or self-indulgent. It may be hard for you to trust.
- 2. Your road to fulfillment requires privacy and the chance to look below the surface. You need to experience intensity, play with power, and to not be shamed.
- An ideal date is watching a sunset together over the ocean, dancing together at a dance or club, or a quiet meal where you can get to know each other.
- Your possible roadblocks to connection include being: withdrawn, power hungry, suspicious, jealous, or shut down if you are made to feel ashamed. You can go wrong by using someone.
- 3. Your road to fulfillment requires intuitive connection, kindness, sensitivity, creativity, and shared trance-like states.
- Your ideal date might be star gazing or sitting quietly before a fire. It might involve a drumming circle, hula hooping, or a candlelit dinner.
- Your possible roadblocks to connection include: being spacey, shy, prone to addictions, delusions, poor judgments, and setting poor boundaries.

As you develop into a sexual being, you will meet partners with different styles. Trying out new styles of expression or blending your style with a partner's can be a source of fun and enjoyment. Your communication style, temperament, and personality will further shape how your sexual nature is expressed. All of these approaches and any combination of these styles are NORMAL. Knowing your inner Venus will help you avoid roadblocks and follow the high road on the journey to becoming a sexual being.

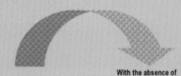

Optimal Male Sexual Response Cycle

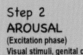

Step 2 AROUSAL
(Excitation phase)
Visual stimuli, genital contact, dreams or fantasy stimulate libido.

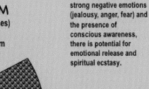

Step 3 ORGASM
(Plateau and orgasm phases) Genital contact for a few minutes will lead to orgasm phase.

With the absence of strong negative emotions (jealousy, anger, fear) and the presence of conscious awareness, there is potential for emotional release and spiritual ecstasy.

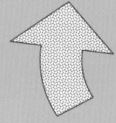

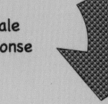

Step 1 DESIRE
Testosterone may be 1000x greater then a female partner.

Step 4 RELAXATION

(Resolution phase) After orgasm many men are relaxed and enjoy sleep.

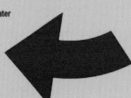

5. Learn about the normal ways men's and women's sexual response cycles differ

FEMALE

Optimal Female Sexual Response Cycle

Step 1 WILLINGNESS

Step 2 RECEPTIVITY
Relationship and environmental factors conducive to being present and open to the sensual imagination and the partner (the absence of fatigue, pain, fear, anger, shame, or guilt) are needed. Delightful sensory experiences are also helpful. The sense of smell is very important to women.

Step 3 OUTERCOURSE
(Excitation phase) Non genital touch with the opportunity for intimate communication and fantasy can lead to heightened sensitivity, pleasure, and lubrication.

Step 4 AROUSAL
(Plateau phase) Once lubrication starts, clitoral stimulation leads to arousal which stimulates feelings of increased libido, decreased modesty, and increased openness to trying new things.

Step 6 RELAXATION (Resolution phase)
After orgasm many women are energized and enjoy processing their feelings. Sharing increases feelings of **INTIMACY**. Leading to greater...

Step 5 ORGASM (Orgasm phase)
Continuous clitoral stimulation, for 20 minutes on average, may be needed for climax to occur. Emotional release, sexual and or spiritual ecstasy also possible.

Often in movies, erotic literature, and especially Internet porn, the focus is completely on vaginal penetration. For men that is often the peak sexual experience. However, only about 15% of all women reach orgasm through vaginal penetration alone and this information is often surprising to inexperienced lovers. It is helpful to realize the difference in the normal male and female sexual response curves. Then you don't have to compare your normal needs and desires with the media version.

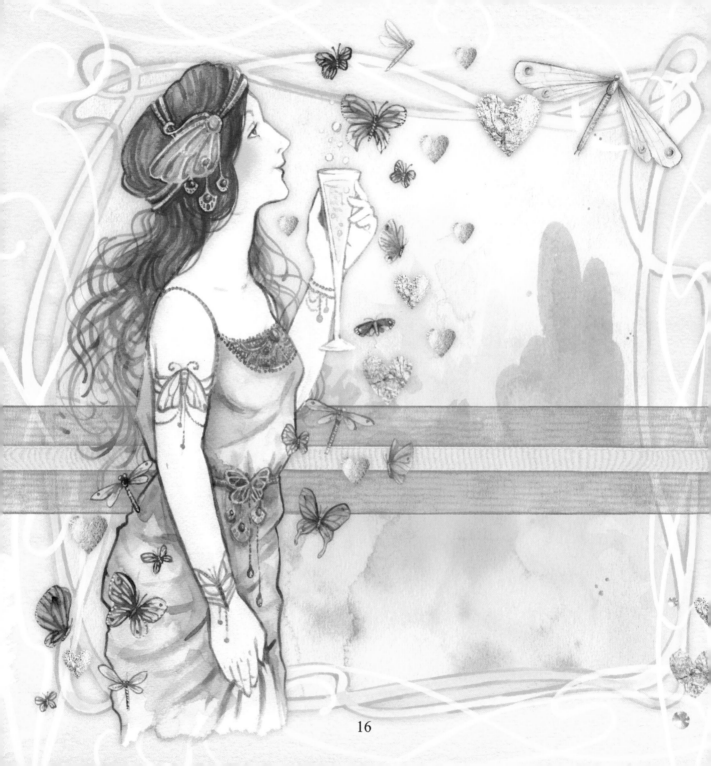

6. Experience Self-pleasuring

If you feel ready to try genital touching, then now is a good time to learn about what feels good to you and learn about how to experience an orgasm. The easiest way to do this may be through teaching yourself by using either your hands or a vibrator. Many women find it easier to experience orgasm through masturbation because no one is watching or judging them. It can be easier to experiment with pleasure on your own, as nothing is off limits, and you may feel more comfortable losing a little control.

Locate your clitoris (see illustration on the next page): it is the center of sexual pleasure for women. Sometimes it helps to look at your genitals in the mirror. The clitoris is near the top of the vulva where the labia meet. Women's labia come in a wide variety of different sizes and shapes. Most labia are not symmetrical. They normally grow after puberty. If you have questions about your body, your health care provider can provide answers.

Touching your clitoris by stroking, rocking, rubbing in circles, or tapping can lead to feeling turned on as blood flows into the area and the clitoris becomes firm and erect. As your sexual response builds, the genitals swell and become wet with a clear vaginal discharge that has a faint scent, and the pelvic floor muscles contract. Massaging the vulva, inner vagina (see illustration), thighs, and or breasts can increase pleasure and can heighten your sensitivity. Some people find viewing erotic art, reading sexually stimulating literature, or imagining a sexually thrilling scenario, increases excitement. Use of a lubricant (such as the paraben free Good Clean Love oil, coconut oil, or aloe gel) or a vibrator can add to the pleasure of the self-experience.

After several times using these techniques, you may come (have an orgasm). This experience is a sudden pleasurable release of sexual tension accompanied by rhythmic pelvic muscle contractions and relaxations. You may find yourself perspiring, moaning, rolling around, rocking your pelvis, arching your back, or just letting go of control of your judging mind and focusing your awareness totally on your pleasant sensual experience. Finding time to pleasure yourself when you can have privacy is good because you are then free to take time, make noise, and be more expressive.

Find the Clitoris

The Vulva

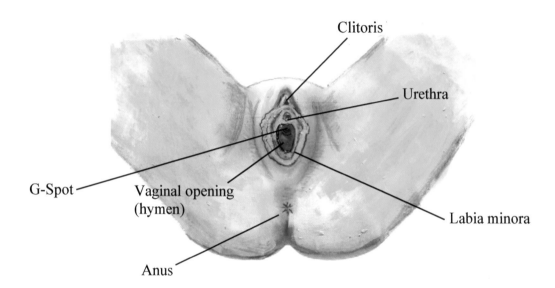

Clitoris

Urethra

G-Spot

Vaginal opening
(hymen)

Labia minora

Anus

Masturbation is a healthy and natural way to help you develop into a sexual being. With experience and experimentation you will find other areas that feel good to touch. The upper front wall of the vagina where the Gspot is located, about 1.5-2 inches inside, is one such erogenous zone. If you would like more information on technique, the book and companion video "Becoming Orgasmic: A Sexual and Personal Growth Program for Women" by Julia Heiman is a great resource. Once you know what feels good to you, it is much easier to express this to your partner when you are together. If self-stimulation is not comfortable for you, your partner can help you have an orgasm. Sharing this information with him or her might be helpful.

7. Set the ground rules
SEX SHOULD BE SAFE!

Before moving on to genital contact with your partner, it is important to agree on the ground rules. Prior to having sex, it helps to agree to what extent you and your partner will keep intimacy confidential, what boundaries you want to set at each point regarding sexual experiences, how you will stay safe (prevent harm), and what each of you would like to receive from the experience. It also helps to be able to discuss how you feel emotionally with your partner and know that your feelings will be respected. You may have spiritual beliefs about sex you would like to discuss. You may want to share this book with your partner as a way to begin this discussion. If your partner does not have a lot of experience he/she may be happy to have a chance to discuss concerns as well.

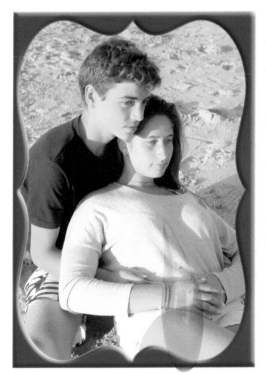

It is important to have up front and frank discussions with your partner about monogamy (whether or not you plan on seeing just each other) and whether or not either of you have a history of sexually transmitted infections. **These discussions require courage but can prevent problems down the road.**

Safety is the most important ground rule. For sex to be safe both you and your partner need to give consent, a clear and enthusiastic "yes" to sexual activity. Consent also includes agreement about protection from sexually transmitted infections and unwanted pregnancy, and this needs to be in place prior to moving forward.

Ideally your partner will have a similar maturity level to your own; this does not necessarily mean you will be of the same age. Every state has its own set of laws about the age at which you can legally consent to sexual activity. Even if sex is agreed to by both people willingly, depending on your age, the state you live in may not consider sexual activity legal. This should be something you think about together when making your decisions about moving forward in a sexual relationship.

Sex involves sharing power and control of another person's pleasure. Set your pace together, talking intimately about what you each want to try and/or what feels good. **There should be positive agreement and understanding at each stage of each sexual encounter to prevent harm. The absence of "no" should not be understood to mean it is okay to proceed.** Make boundaries clear, and be sure you both know it is important to communicate before going further. Each time you are together genital contact should happen by mutual agreement. Just because you have done something once, it does not mean you are necessarily ready to do it the next time.

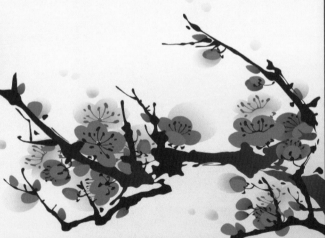

The use of alcohol or drugs can seriously interfere with your judgment about whether you want to have sex. It can also impair your partner's judgment. The majority of date rape (sexual assault by an intimate partner) involves drugs and alcohol. So try to avoid sexual situations where you and/or your partner are not able to make good decisions. Sexual assault occurs when a person forcefully touches another person in an attempt to obtain sexual satisfaction without the victim's conscious and voluntary consent. If you feel you are in danger of being sexually assaulted you should leave or call 911. If you have been assaulted, call your physician, law enforcement, or have a family member or trusted friend take you to your nearest emergency room.

Just because someone takes you out on a date or buys you something, you are not obligated to have sex with them.
You are never obligated to have sex with anyone.

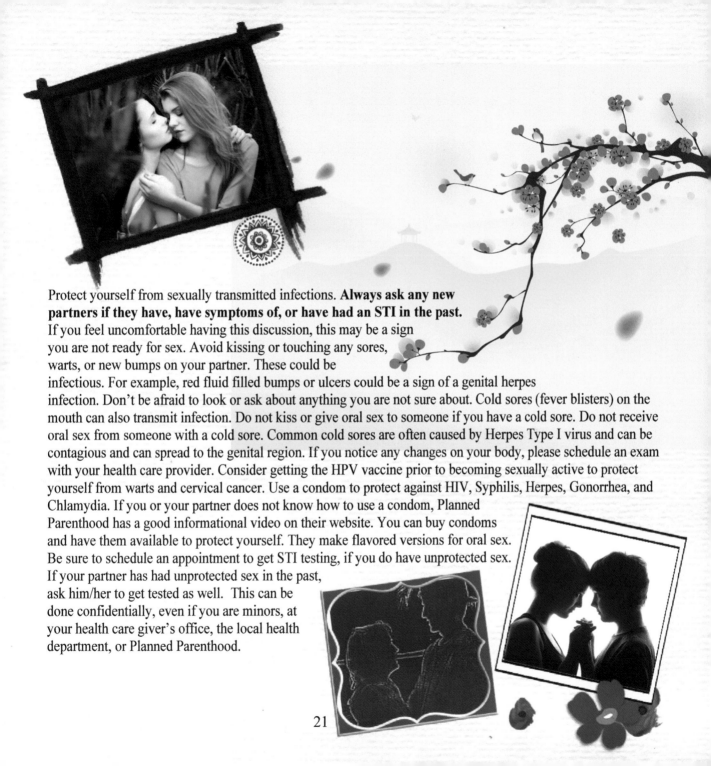

Protect yourself from sexually transmitted infections. **Always ask any new partners if they have, have symptoms of, or have had an STI in the past.** If you feel uncomfortable having this discussion, this may be a sign you are not ready for sex. Avoid kissing or touching any sores, warts, or new bumps on your partner. These could be infectious. For example, red fluid filled bumps or ulcers could be a sign of a genital herpes infection. Don't be afraid to look or ask about anything you are not sure about. Cold sores (fever blisters) on the mouth can also transmit infection. Do not kiss or give oral sex to someone if you have a cold sore. Do not receive oral sex from someone with a cold sore. Common cold sores are often caused by Herpes Type I virus and can be contagious and can spread to the genital region. If you notice any changes on your body, please schedule an exam with your health care provider. Consider getting the HPV vaccine prior to becoming sexually active to protect yourself from warts and cervical cancer. Use a condom to protect against HIV, Syphilis, Herpes, Gonorrhea, and Chlamydia. If you or your partner does not know how to use a condom, Planned Parenthood has a good informational video on their website. You can buy condoms and have them available to protect yourself. They make flavored versions for oral sex. Be sure to schedule an appointment to get STI testing, if you do have unprotected sex. If your partner has had unprotected sex in the past, ask him/her to get tested as well. This can be done confidentially, even if you are minors, at your health care giver's office, the local health department, or Planned Parenthood.

21

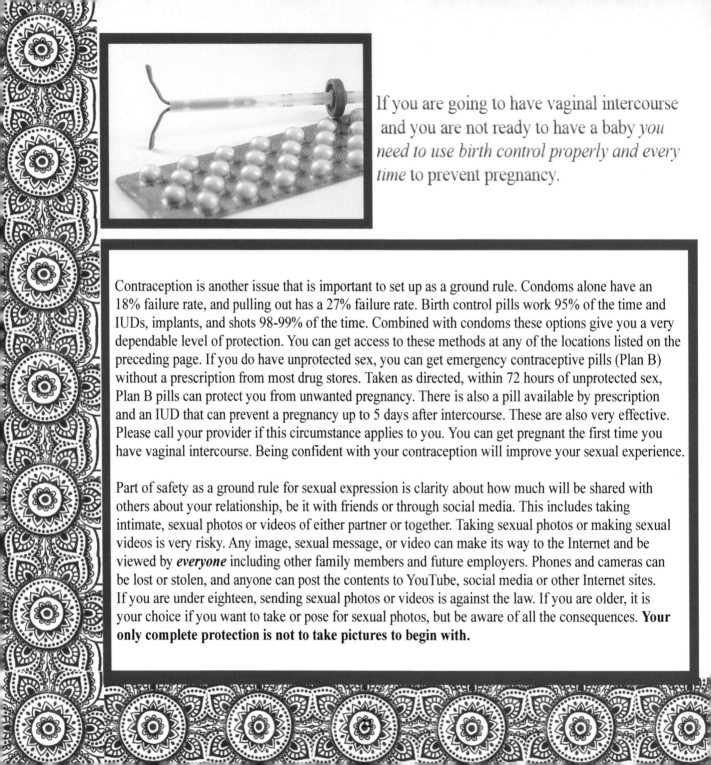

If you are going to have vaginal intercourse and you are not ready to have a baby *you need to use birth control properly and every time* to prevent pregnancy.

Contraception is another issue that is important to set up as a ground rule. Condoms alone have an 18% failure rate, and pulling out has a 27% failure rate. Birth control pills work 95% of the time and IUDs, implants, and shots 98-99% of the time. Combined with condoms these options give you a very dependable level of protection. You can get access to these methods at any of the locations listed on the preceding page. If you do have unprotected sex, you can get emergency contraceptive pills (Plan B) without a prescription from most drug stores. Taken as directed, within 72 hours of unprotected sex, Plan B pills can protect you from unwanted pregnancy. There is also a pill available by prescription and an IUD that can prevent a pregnancy up to 5 days after intercourse. These are also very effective. Please call your provider if this circumstance applies to you. You can get pregnant the first time you have vaginal intercourse. Being confident with your contraception will improve your sexual experience.

Part of safety as a ground rule for sexual expression is clarity about how much will be shared with others about your relationship, be it with friends or through social media. This includes taking intimate, sexual photos or videos of either partner or together. Taking sexual photos or making sexual videos is very risky. Any image, sexual message, or video can make its way to the Internet and be viewed by *everyone* including other family members and future employers. Phones and cameras can be lost or stolen, and anyone can post the contents to YouTube, social media or other Internet sites. If you are under eighteen, sending sexual photos or videos is against the law. If you are older, it is your choice if you want to take or pose for sexual photos, but be aware of all the consequences. **Your only complete protection is not to take pictures to begin with.**

Setting the ground rules and creating a safe sexual environment takes courage, but it is a very important part of developing trust in each relationship.

Open and honest discussions with a potential sexual partner will get easier each time you see how your conversations increase intimacy and decrease heartbreak. Being able to speak openly and honestly is a skill that will benefit you throughout your lifetime. An open channel of communication between you and your partner before sex will make it much easier to talk during sex. In the beginning, no one is an expert. So being able to ask questions like "does this feel good" or give directions such as "slower" or "go deeper" will help you gain knowledge, understand each other better, and be better lovers.

As you both learn to please each other, your sexual relationship will evolve and deepen. For a female to have the healthiest and most fulfilling sexual response, the relationship needs to be one of mutual respect, trust, kindness, and open communication. First sexual experiences should not be something you regret, but instead be the satisfying experience of two consenting individuals gaining a shared experience of pleasure in a kind and loving way. By laying this foundation for sexual experiencing, no matter what happens in the future with your relationship, you will maintain your self-respect, your respect for your partner, and positive feelings about sex.

What are your thoughts about confidentiality, monogamy, and safety? How far do you want to go at this point with trying new things? Where are your boundaries?

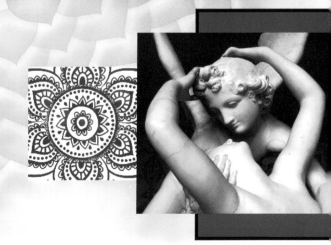

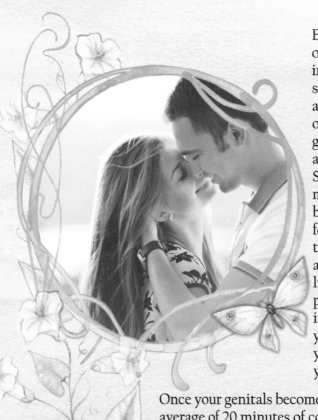

Experiencing intimate genital contact and having orgasms with your partner without vaginal intercourse is a further step on your journey of sexual unfolding. Use the knowledge you gained about what turns you on and how to have an orgasm to help your partner understand what feels good to you. Likewise, you can ask your partner about what type of genital touch he/she likes. Start with nongenital sexual play for at least 10 to 15 minutes before genital contact. This allows you to become aroused with your whole body. It allows for a heightening of your senses, it gives your body time to make hormones that enhance the experience, and it allows you to begin to lubricate. Once lubrication occurs, genital touching is more pleasurable. If your partner is not very experienced, it is helpful to show him/her how you like to have your genitals touched and where your clitoris is. Let your partner know that for comfort and pleasure, your genitals must be lubricated before any touch.

Once your genitals become wet and you are moderately aroused, it takes an average of 20 minutes of continuous clitoral contact for you to become aroused enough to have an orgasm. This is normal for women and is different from a man's quicker arousal cycle (See Step 5).

8. Try genital touch and orgasm with a partner

Kissing, licking, or sucking a partner's genital area is referred to as oral sex. You may hear other terms for oral sex. Cunnilingus is the oral pleasuring of a woman's clitoris, vagina, or vulva by her partner's lips and tongue. The term "blow job" is slang for fellatio, which is the male equivalent. It is stimulation of a man's penis, scrotum or perineum by his partner's mouth, usually by licking or sucking. There is no blowing involved. Oral sex is one way to bring a partner to orgasm.

If you have an orgasm by manual or oral stimulation, in addition to the physical release of muscle tension, 5-15% of women ejaculate (release) fluid from the vagina with orgasm. If your male partner is having an orgasm too, when he ejaculates there may be a lot of seminal fluid as well. Sometimes it is helpful to have a small towel or washcloth available to dry off with after sex. It is ok to have sex during your period if you are in the mood and if you are not having too many menstrual cramps. Menstrual blood is a normal bodily fluid like semen or vaginal lubrication.

With orgasm, some people experience an emotional release as well, with tears or laughter. These are all normal occurrences. Often having orgasms with your partner without vaginal intercourse can help trust and understanding grow. Sometimes you may come (have an orgasm) first, sometimes your partner will, sometimes you may reach climax together. Hopefully, each time together, both partners will have the opportunity to feel desire, pleasure, and satisfaction.

It may take a number of times together before your partner discovers the type of touching and kissing that makes you come. So don't worry if this does not happen right away. Sexual satisfaction can mean different things to different people depending on each person's motivations. For some people their greatest enjoyment comes from the feelings of love or connection. Others value the post sexual feeling of oneness and peace. Orgasm is a pleasurable experience but does not need to be considered the sole goal for sexual satisfaction. It is simply part of becoming a sexual being. Sexual fulfillment is necessary for continued interest and enjoyment in sex. Enjoy your time discovering what brings you and your partner satisfaction.

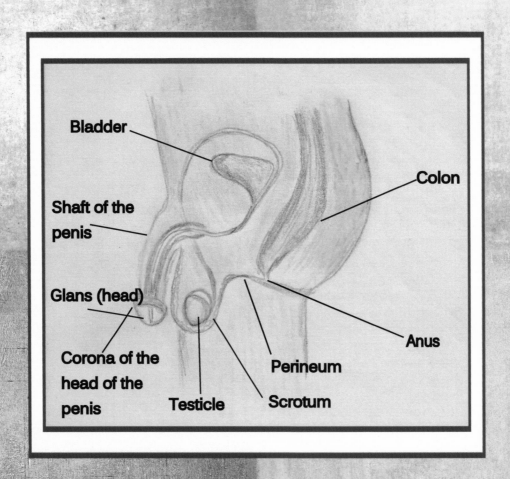

Bladder

Colon

Shaft of the
penis

Glans (head)

Corona of the
head of the
penis

Testicle

Perineum

Scrotum

Anus

26

If you have a female partner, you will be able to be intuitive about what might feel good to her. If you have a male partner you may be curious about how to touch his genitals. First you should ask your partner if they would like you to touch them. It is also ok to ask him to tell you or show you how he likes to be touched. Some of the ways to pleasurably touch the penis include: wrapping your fingers around the shaft and moving your hand up and down in a slow, steady motion, or you can use two hands in the same or opposite directions. You can also vary your speed and pressure. Other touches that may be pleasurable include: stroking the corona (the rim where the head meets the shaft) massaging, cupping, or gently patting the the scrotum, or massaging the perineum (area between the anus and testicles). Your partner may have been circumcised as a child, this is a religious and/or cultural procedure where the foreskin is removed from the glans of the penis. If your partner is not circumcised, he will have skin that slides over the glans. When touching your partner, pay attention to his body language to see if what you are doing brings a positive response. For most men, the penis will become firm and hard (erect) with pleasurable touch. Further stimulation will lead to ejaculation, orgasm, and release of semen. Semen is a collection of sperm and fluid. Men cannot urinate while ejaculating.

9. VAGINAL INTERCOURSE

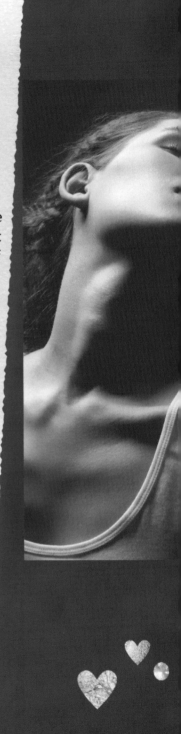

Sex is a whole body, whole person experience. If you are in a heterosexual relationship, at some point in your sexual life you may want to experience vaginal intercourse. There are several things you can do to make the first time enjoyable. The vaginal opening with its surrounding fringe of tissue(hymen) is smaller prior to vaginal intercourse, so prior to the first time, you can gently stretch the vaginal opening, hymen, and vaginal muscles. All muscles can lengthen and become more elastic with gentle stretching. If you are already comfortable using tampons, this will be fairly easy.

The vaginal walls are made of muscles that gradually lengthen with stretching, just like your hamstrings do when you stretch or do yoga. Your vaginal opening will gradually become more flexible with stretching and other activities (e.g., jumping on a trampoline, horseback riding, playing sports, vaginal intercourse, and childbirth). If you have not stretched and warmed up the vaginal muscles beforehand, when you first have intercourse it is possible you may bleed a little.

You can prepare your vagina for intercourse by stretching in the shower or bath or the privacy of your room. Using a water-based or oil based lubricant like Good Clean Love or the original K-Y jelly, introduce one finger into the vagina and gently stretch the muscles. You should particularly press toward the perineum (back wall of the vagina above the anus) rather than stretching side to side. On subsequent sessions introduce more fingers as the stretch becomes comfortable until you can comfortably insert three fingers. Using a small water proof vibrator is another way to massage and gently dilate the vagina.

When you stretch the muscles you can also play with contracting and relaxing the muscles around your fingers. This is the Kegel exercise. Contracting and relaxing your pelvic floor muscles can increase pleasure once you begin to have intercourse.

Your partner can stretch your vagina as well. By touching and gently stretching the vagina during love-making, as described previously, he will become aware of your vaginal size and shape. This knowledge can help him realize how your bodies may fit together. You should be able to comfortably allow two or three fingers before proceeding to intercourse. It could take a couple of weeks to reach enough familiarity for this to be comfortable. While many couples have quite a bit of touch experience, some couples come together for the first time on their wedding night and have no experience. *Vaginal intercourse should not be attempted until the hymeneal opening and vagina can comfortably accommodate an erect penis.*

In the beginning, have intercourse when you are most turned on immediately after or just before *you* orgasm. Vaginal penetration is easiest when you are at the peak of arousal because the vagina is wet and dilated. At this point, the tissues are also supported by the increased blood flow. Do not wait too long after orgasm. Within a few minutes after orgasm you enter the resolution (relaxation) phase of the sexual response cycle (see Step 5) and your tissues can be more fragile and prone to tearing or discomfort. If you have not yet had an orgasm, begin vaginal intercourse when you are very aroused as evidenced by your own natural vaginal lubrication. At this point you may also notice your pulse racing, your labia swelling and deepening in color, your body breaking out in a thin layer of sweat, and your clitoris becoming firm and erect. Those are all normal sensations. If you do have an orgasm you will notice rhythmic contractions of the genitals and pelvic muscles. Even though you may feel very aroused and wet, it is still a good idea to use a lubricant in the beginning. This will allow a smoother sliding in and decrease friction from the condom. Use a good water based lubricant (such as Good Clean Love gel). **Oil based lubricants break down latex condoms so avoid them for vaginal intercourse when you plan to use a condom.** Alternatively you can buy lubricated condoms.

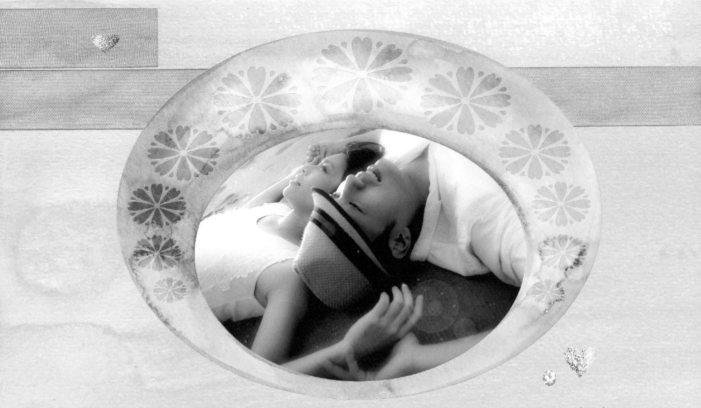

The first time you have vaginal intercourse, your partner should enter your vagina slowly, completely, and then rest. Be sure the labia minora (see illustration) are open and not pulled into the vagina. You need time to relax and let yourself feel his penis inside. If you need to move to adjust things for comfort, do so. Guys will feel an urge to move back and forth, so communicate before and during sex about how slow to go.

You can rest together in stillness while kissing or talking. Most of the time, this will be enough for the first experience. Gentle slow pelvic movements are better in the beginning. After a few minutes if it becomes uncomfortable plan to stop and have orgasm together a different way. In the future, more vigorous pelvic thrusting can be attempted as you become more comfortable. It is not normal to have pain with sex. *If you experience pain in the vulva, vagina, or abdomen during intercourse, you should stop. You can try a different position, but if that does not help, you should see a health care provider for an exam to determine the cause.* Trauma and pain can cause fear and increased muscle tension in the future, so it's important that this first experience be as pain-free and enjoyable as possible.

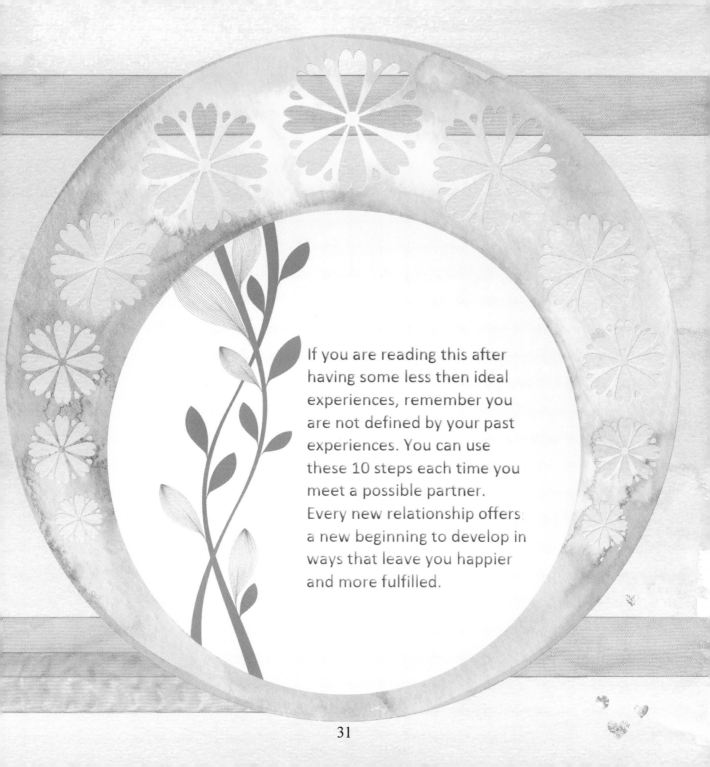

If you are reading this after having some less then ideal experiences, remember you are not defined by your past experiences. You can use these 10 steps each time you meet a possible partner. Every new relationship offers a new beginning to develop in ways that leave you happier and more fulfilled.

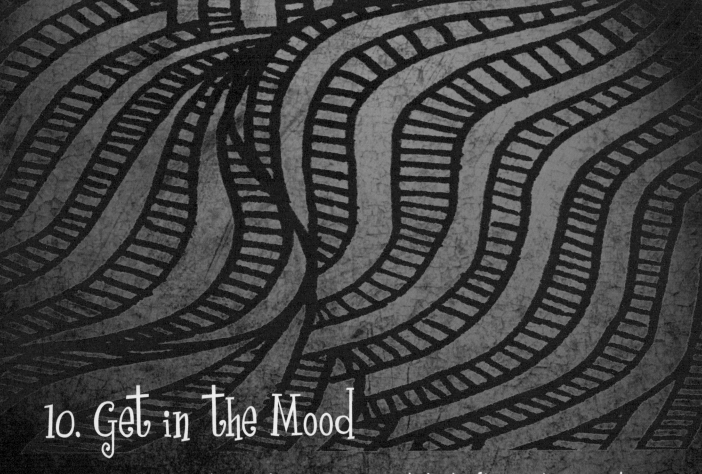

10. Get in the Mood

Early in relationships, when people are new to sex, desire is often spontaneous and strong due to novelty, attraction, and higher hormone levels. However, when you first become sexually active you may feel a bit unsure about your sexual inexperience. Worries or other distraction may make it hard to get in the mood. There are several things you can do to help with this. First, create a space that allows for privacy, sensuality, and the opportunity to focus on each other without interruption. You want to have a private place where you can spend time together, focusing only on each other.

When you are experiencing and giving pleasure you want to be able to let the sensual imagination run free without worries, intrusions or electronic devices. Locking doors and turning off or silencing cell phones makes for a better sexual experience.

Pay attention to lighting, textures, sounds, and scents. A woman's sexual response is very affected by her sense of smell. Consider lighting scented candles, or bringing flowers into the room. When you are first starting out, you may not have a lot of options for places to be together, but you can start with simple suggestions and advance from there. For example, showering or bathing before lovemaking creates a more appealing atmosphere.

Sexual desire is often stimulated by visual cues. These can include dimming the lights or getting dressed up for a date. Textures and fabrics that feel good on the skin or lingerie may also help create a sensual environment. Only do what adds to your own enjoyment and personal sense of attractiveness. Some people like the feeling of trimming or removing leg or pubic hair, other people find a natural hair pattern more pleasing to them. Give some consideration to what feels good to you. Playing music is another simple way to convey a message to yourself and your partner that you are ready to move from the more everyday world to the sensuous world.

What ideas do you have about creating a sexual space you would feel comfortable in?

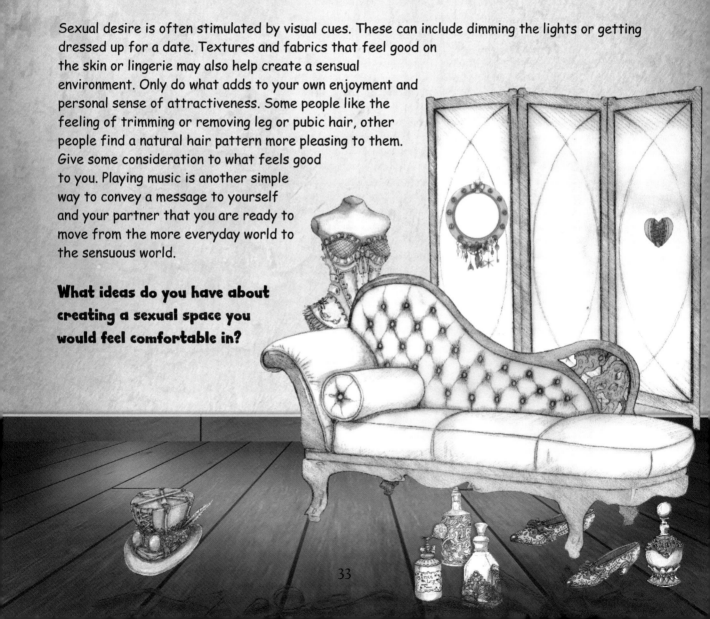

33

After you have created a sensual outer space you may need to shift your inner frame of mind as well. If the mind is busy thinking about other things, or worrying, it can be difficult to feel desire or become aroused. Worries, especially those related to sexual "performance" can really be a turn off. It is just as important to good sex to turn off your worries as it is to turn off your cell phone. Negativity in general (jealousy, anger, fear, shame, guilt) can all interfere with opening your heart and connecting with your partner on an emotional and spiritual level.

Sexual desire flows more easily when you are physically fit and well rested. Your desire hormone (testosterone) peaks in the morning after a good night's sleep. Getting regular moderate exercise and plenty of sleep makes it easier to get in the mood. This will help your own spontaneous healthy sexual desire flow.

Desire also grows when you are "present in the moment" with an open heart. This means your attention is focused on what is happening in the present moment with yourself and your partner. To help you stay focused and turn your thoughts away from distractions it is helpful to focus on your breathing and bring your attention to how you are feeling. You can slowly check your mental, physical, emotional, and energetic states. To do this you can start by breathing consciously for a few breaths. Notice how active your mind is: if your thinking mind begins to wander or it feels agitated, ask it to calm down. Bring your focus back on your breath and then start to notice how your physical body is feeling. By moving through your body, contracting and relaxing your muscles from head to toe you can become more present. This technique is called Progressive Muscle Relaxation. It can help you relax and calm the mind. There are many relaxation techniques and examples available online. (UNH Health Services has a good YouTube video demonstrating Progressive Muscle Relaxation.)

Looking deeply into each other's eyes when you are both present in the moment is a uniquely human joy.

Next, survey your senses. Opening our awareness to sensual pleasure gets libido going. Notice what you can hear, smell, and taste in this moment. Open up to any tactile sensation you feel such as cool, soft, or smooth. See if you can feel acceptance and appreciation for your physical body.

Once you are focused and "present" in your physical body, move on to your emotional body. Try to pick up on whatever emotional state is present and take it in. Notice how it feels to be you in your heart. If you feel fearful, what does that feel like? What does excited feel like? Whatever mood you perceive, open your heart, breathe in, and accept yourself. When this happens, you create a positive and loving environment for yourself and your partner.

Finally, tune into your energetic body. Observe how alive you feel and if you can, use your breath to bring a sense of energy to your entire body. Connecting to your vitality can energize your lovemaking. Sometimes you might try lying next to your partner and breathing together or breathing together while you look into each other's eyes. Relaxing your mind and being open and present will allow you to fully feel each sensual pleasure. Being conscious and aware of your partner's responses to your touch and your partner's emotional and energetic state will also improve your connection to your partner. Looking deeply and lovingly into each other's eyes when you are truly present with each other is a uniquely human joy.

If you have an active mind, you can practice your focused breathing and connecting to the present moment throughout the day, especially when there is something you find pleasurable, like a vivid color, a delicious taste, a cool breeze. Nature is especially helpful. Walking in a flower scented meadow, swimming in the moonlight, or just getting outside can take you away from all your thoughts and worries. Imagine your favorite tastes, scents and textures; how does this make you feel, can you feel your sensual energy flowing? Take a moment and open your sensual awareness and your body to each opportunity.

35

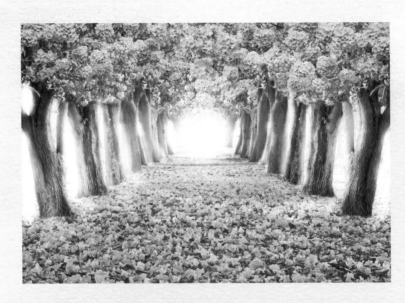

Closing

Becoming a sexual being is a lifelong journey. On this journey, you will cross one-way thresholds of knowing. This journey should therefore be taken with care. Consider carefully each step of the journey, use this book as a guide, and find a supportive person to talk to about any questions or concerns you have.

Take time to discover when you are ready, follow your own path, set the ground rules, play, get to know your inner "Venus," experience self-pleasuring, learn about the normal ways men's and women's sexual response cycles differ, and get in the mood. Try genital touch and orgasm with a partner, and have vaginal intercourse in a planned and conscious way.

Pleasure, knowledge, and intimacy with a partner are the gifts of this type of exploration. Intimacy is sharing a deep understanding, affection, and familiarity with another human being. As you open yourself up to your partner sexually, you allow him/her to see, touch, and physically enter your body. You can become unselfconscious and at ease together. When you both accept and appreciate each other physically in non-judgmental ways, intimacy begins.

Emotional intimacy develops as each person risks sharing something that reveals something about their deepest dreams, secrets, and desires. When you discover and reveal something important about yourself and your partner receives that in a loving, accepting way, an emotional bond is formed. Then it is your partner's turn to take you into their confidence. If each of you is able to do this with a loving heart and open mind, a deeper more meaningful bond grows. Each time that you share feelings openly, you deepen emotional intimacy. Trust grows when you reciprocate and honor each other's feelings.

With mental intimacy you share your thoughts, beliefs, and ideas. You start to share inner jokes and memories. With a committed partner you may find unconscious, unresolved issues come to the surface to be worked on together. An intimate partner can be the only one who may help you get clarity and work on roadblocks you might have with things like trust, abandonment, honesty, repressed emotions, etc.

Over your sexual lifetime you may have the opportunity to develop spiritual intimacy with a person. You can begin to communicate with a look, end each other's sentences, and know what each other is thinking. This usually happens after many months to years of respect, trust, and love. You may become able to experience spiritual ecstasy together. By looking into each other's eyes, while being completely present in intense passion, you can expand with your partner into a greater wholeness.

The journey to the sexual universe,
when explored in a conscious way,
can be full of pleasure, understanding, joy, and deep bonding.
Bon voyage!

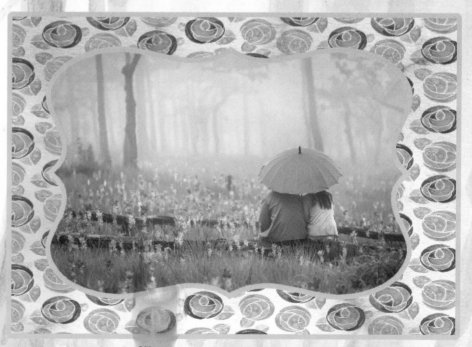

Glossary of terms

Abstinent: Not sexually active.

Arousal: Sexual stimulation, excitement or response.

Bisexual: A person sexually attracted to both men and women.

Blow job: A slang term for *fellatio*, or the stimulation of a man's penis, scrotum or perineum by his partner's mouth, usually by licking or sucking.

Consensual: Agreed to and willingly participated in by the people involved.

Contraception: A technique or practice used to prevent pregnancy.

Contraceptive: A device or drug used to prevent pregnancy.

Cunnilingus: The oral pleasuring of a woman's clitoris, vagina, or vulva by her partner's lips and tongue.

Date rape: Sexual assault by an intimate partner.

Ejaculate: Release.

Erogenous zones: Parts of the human body that are more highly sensitive to and respond to sexual stimulation.

Feel the wanting: Experiencing desire in a slow and deliberate way.

Fellatio: *See* Blow job.

Genital: Relating to the sexual organs.

Inner Venus: Your sexual self, comprised of what you find attractive, your style of attracting partners, how you find fulfillment on your sexual journey and your roadblocks to fulfillment.

Lesbian: A woman whose emotional and sexual energies are geared towards other women.

Libido: Sexual desire.

Masturbation: The stimulation of one's own genitals for the purpose of sexual arousal.

Monogamy: The practice of having a sexual relationship with just one partner.

Oral sex: Kissing, licking or sucking a partner's genital area.

Orgasm: The peak or point of greatest sexual intensity and excitement also referred to as climax.

Outercourse: Sexual stimulation that does not include genital contact.

Pelvic floor muscles: The muscles that support the pelvis and pelvic organs.

Perineum: A region of the body located between the vagina and anus in females and scrotum and anus in males.

Progressive muscle relaxation: A relaxation technique and process that involves relaxing muscle groups.

Resolution: Relaxation where the body returns to its normal levels of function/feeling.

Semen, seminal fluid: Fluid produced by the male's sexual organs.

Sexual: Relating to sex; relating to the instincts, physiological processes, and activities connected with physical attraction or physical intimacy.

Sexual assault: When a person forcefully touches another person as an attempt to obtain sexual satisfaction without the victim's conscious and voluntary consent.

Sexual being: The part of being human that involves the desire for sexual exploration and gratification, acceptance by others, self-acceptance, and relationship development.

Straight (Heterosexual): A person attracted to people of the opposite sex or gender.

Acknowledgments

In the past few years, many of my patients have sent their daughters to me at the cusp of sexuality for counseling and health care. I am so grateful for the trust they have placed in me, and this book has arisen in response to that need. Laurie Watson, LMFT, LPC, a well-known local sex therapist, speaking at a continuing education conference, shared some concerning research findings. In the US, more than half of males surveyed ranked their First Sexual Initiation (FSI) encounters as positive, while more than half of US females had negative feelings about their FSI. In one study 1/3 of the females described their FSI as disappointing or disastrous. Her talk motivated me to do something to improve this situation. Laurie kindly shared background information from her website that got me started on this project. After reading a study that showed that **in females, positive responses to FSI were associated with planning of the FSI, longer relationships with the partner, contraception use, positive body image, and positive messages about sex,** I decided to focus on steps to help achieve a positive experience.

The work of Gina Ogden and the Isis Survey fell in with the approach I normally take with patients and helped me form a framework. The lectures I attended by Steven Forest entitled "Love and Mischief" helped me better understand the psychological and spiritual aspects of intimacy development. The stories and ideas of many friends further informed this work. I would like to thank Lizzette Potthoff, Brooke Ferrell, Amy and Erin McCormack, Beth Posner, Samantha Brody, SaraJo Berman, Kate Dunn, Mark Dellavalle, and Emily and Natalia Motyka. I would especially like to thank Rachel Anderson, Sex Education Teacher at Carolina Friends School, for her reading and helpful editorial suggestions. Laurie Lindgren gave me the complete support I needed to follow my own path. She contributed many wonderful suggestions. My friend Lauren Winslow was completely vital in getting me to think out of the traditional medical box. Her careful reading, editing, and hours discussing ideas with me were absolutely invaluable. Lucie Branham, generous friend and careful editor, was integral to the project. She devoted countless hours to helping me make the ideas into a user friendly and practical guide. Her backing allowed me to follow my vision and begin and end with the same enthusiasm. I could not have done it without her! I would like to thank Tom Motyka, my husband, for his patience and support for this project, for discussing with me and helping me as I worked through each step. Finally I would like to acknowledge Jolan, our daughter. This book is for you, my dear, and all women like you starting out on this journey.

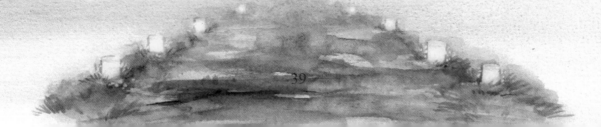

CPSIA information can be obtained at www.ICGtesting.com
Printed in the USA
BVIW12n2028200915
418222BV00017B/113

* 9 7 8 0 6 9 2 3 8 8 5 9 4 *